First published 2012 by Pearson Education Limited

Published 2014 by Routledge

2 Park Square, Milton Park, Abingdon, Oxon OX14 4RN

711 Third Avenue, New York, NY 10017, USA

Routledge is an imprint of the Taylor & Francis Group, an informa business

Copyright © 2012, Taylor & Francis.

The right of Nina Godson to be identified as author of this work has been
asserted by her in accordance with the Copyright, Designs and Patents Act 1988.

ISBN 13: 978-0-273-73897-8 (hbk)

British Library Cataloguing-in-Publication Data
A catalogue record for this book is available from the British Library

Library of Congress Cataloging-in-Publication Data
A catalog record for this book is av

Typeset in 8/9.5pt Helvetica by 35

Printed in the UK by Severn,

Paper
respon
FSC®
www.fsc.org

T0298274

contents

The assessment of clinical skills competencies is an essential element of the educational process in any health care training and the safety of patients in the clinical environment. Objective structured clinical examinations (OSCE) are one form of assessment, used as both formative and summative assessment, which identifies objective performance criteria for the clinical skill being examined, for example hand-washing steps.

■ WHAT IS AN OBJECTIVE STRUCTURED CLINICAL EXAMINATION?

An OSCE is an examination used to assess and test clinical skills performance and competence, increasingly used in health care professions training, such as nursing, midwifery, operating departmental practice, paramedic science and medicine. This type of clinical examination gives the student the opportunity to be assessed on clinical skills that have been practised in a safe environment, with safe rehearsal. The clinical tutor is able to assess whether the student is safe and competent to attend clinical placement. OSCEs involve the student rotating through one or more practical and theoretical 'stations', where he or she is assessed using a set of criteria, according to the chosen clinical skill.

■ OSCE DESIGN

An OSCE comprises a number of stations that have a particular skill for the student to perform safely. The stations vary in time constraints, according to the level required. Each station has its own examiner and a simulated patient (either an actor or a manikin). Candidates rotate from station to station as directed, or visit one station only.

Objective

All candidates are assessed using the same marking scheme, according to the training establishment and level required. OSCE candidates receive marks for each step of the skill that they perform correctly, therefore making the assessment objective rather than subjective.

Structured

Work stations have very specific tasks. Instructions are written carefully to ensure that the candidate is given a very specific skill to complete. Simulated patients and examiners provide detailed feedback to all candidates on their performance.

Clinical examination

The OSCE is designed to assess clinical and theoretical knowledge, depending on the academic level of the student.

■ OSCE MARKING CRITERIA

Marking is carried out by an examiner and is moderated by an OSCE team, usually comprising the individuals who coordinate and teach the module. One of the ways an OSCE is made objective is by having a detailed marking scheme and a standard set of questions, depending on the level of study. The examiner may vary the marks depending on how well the candidate performs the steps of the clinical skill, but expectations should be agreed beforehand, often through organised meetings. At the end of the mark sheet, the examiner may have a number of marks that they can use to 'weight' the student's performance and verbal presentation. The weighted marks have to be agreed by the OSCE team. A simulated patient may be asked to comment on the student's performance to give the student and examiner insight into the patient's experience. At the end, the examiner is often asked to give a 'global score': the examiner is usually asked to rate the candidate as pass, borderline or fail. Results are not always given immediately.

■ GETTING PREPARED FOR YOUR OSCE

Dress code – be professional!

Wear appropriate clothing, as instructed by your tutor:

- Clean uniform provided by your place of learning
- Flat sensible shoes of the correct colour (for a stable base and safety)
- No jewellery except for a wedding band (in case it gets caught in equipment and for infection-control reasons)
- Hair tied back and off the collar (to prevent the spread of infection)
- Name badge visible (so the examiner and simulated patient can identify you)
- No nail polish or long nails
- Minimal makeup
- Watch with a second hand (to time procedures)
- Black pen (for documentation)

All clinical equipment required to perform the skills should be provided by the establishment. Familiarise yourself with how it works before the OSCE.

The next chapters give examples of OSCE stations. Read the chapters carefully and then practise each clinical skill in a small group within a classroom or skills laboratory or at home. Practice makes perfect!

■ USEFUL TIPS

- In a group of three, one student can be the examiner and use the assessment sheets provided in this book, one student can be the patient, and one student can be the OSCE candidate. Then swap round.
- The skill of the correct hand washing-technique (Ayliffe procedure) should be used at the beginning and at the end of every practical skill and at any other appropriate times during the process.
- It is important that you understand the anatomy and physiology of the body systems related to the clinical skill being examined. Any good anatomy and physiology text such as *Anatomy and Physiology for Nursing and Health Professionals* by Colbert *et al.* (Pearson Education, 2009) should provide you with the detail necessary to fully understand the skill you are undertaking.
- Clinical measurements are also referred to as patient observations or vital signs. Clinical measurements include measuring blood pressure, temperature, pulse and respirations. When undertaking clinical measurements, perception and observation skills should be used alongside knowledge to ensure that any clinical deterioration of the patient is promptly detected, reported, acted upon and recorded.

Infection prevention

■ EQUIPMENT REQUIRED TO WASH HANDS

- Liquid soap
- Hand drier or paper towels

■ WHAT CAN THE SKIN TELL US?

Nutrition status The skin needs to be nourished by the correct nutrients to keep it healthy and supple and enable it to heal efficiently. If the skin is not nourished, it may look dull and dry, break down easily, and take longer to repair.

Fluid balance The skin can become dehydrated if there is insufficient supply of fluid in the diet. One way of testing for dehydrated skin is the pinch test (**to be used only if the patient consents**): gently pinch the skin – if it does not spring back into its normal position, it may mean that the patient is dehydrated.

Blood circulation If the skin has a good supply of oxygen and nutrients, it may look pink and glowing. If circulation is poor, the skin may be blue in colour (cyanosed). Be aware that differently pigmented skins will vary in colour.

Emotional state If the person is anxious or worried, they may sweat.

Age The skin changes with age, for example wrinkles, liver spots and thinning of the skin.

Health problems Skin complaints such as eczema, rashes and steroidal treatment may be obvious.

Evaluation of effectiveness of care If the skin is dirty and unwashed, it may indicate that the person is not taking care of themselves.

■ AIMS OF THE CORRECT HAND-WASHING TECHNIQUE (AYLIFFE PROCEDURE, EIGHT STEPS)

- To ensure hands are free from transient micro-organisms.
- To prevent the transfer of transient micro-organisms from one person to another.
- To reduce the risk of health-care-acquired infection.

■ WHEN SHOULD HANDS BE WASHED?

- After visiting the toilet
- Before eating food
- When hands are visibly soiled
- Before and after each clinical procedure (and sometimes more often if necessary)
- Between caring for different patients (extra precautions may have to be taken if barrier nursing is in place)
- After contact with any bodily fluids, such as urine, faeces, vomit and blood.

■ AYLIFFE PROCEDURE: EIGHT-STEP HAND-WASHING TECHNIQUE

1. Wet hands under running water (use your elbow to turn the tap on if possible). Use one measure of soap. (Remember: it's not the amount of soap you use that is important – it's the rubbing action that removes dead skin cells and micro-organisms).
2. Work soap into hands, palm to palm (five times).
3. Position right hand over back of left, and vice versa (five times).
4. Rub palm to palm, fingers interlaced (five times).
5. Rub back of left fingers to right palm, fingers interlocked, and vice versa (five times).

6. Rotational rubbing of right thumb clasped in left hand, and vice versa (five times).
7. Rub left palm with clasped fingers of right hand, and vice versa (five times).
8. Rub left wrist with right hand, and vice versa (five times).

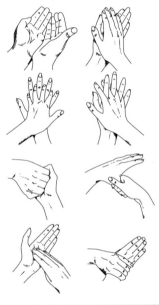

From Ayliffe GAJ, Babb JR, Quoraishi AH (1978) A test for hygienic hand disinfection. *Journal of Clinical Pathology* **31**: 923–28. © BMJ Publishing Group Ltd.

■ TIPS TO SUCCESS IN YOUR OSCE

Communication skills Introduce yourself, stating your role and full name. Ask the patient's name and what they would like to be called.

Equipment Use only the equipment needed (see list above).

Infection prevention Always wash your hands using the Ayliffe procedure at the beginning and at the end of a procedure, and at any other times when necessary.

Results Remember it is not the amount of soap you use but the rubbing action that removes germs.

Use of taps and disposal of hand towels Where possible, use your elbows to turn taps on and off. When disposing of paper towels, use the pedal to avoid touching the bin.

Report If no soap or paper towels are available, report to the appropriate person.

Patient comfort Encourage patients to wash their hands when needed.

Drying hands Take one paper towel and dry in one direction, from the fingertips to the wrist. Do not go back in the same direction as this takes any remaining micro-organisms back up to the hands. Repeat the procedure until the hands and wrists are dry. Use the pedal to open the bin and discard the paper towel.

Hand air-dryer Hands can be dried using a hand air-dryer: ensure your hands are thoroughly dried and do not leave any damp surfaces, where micro-organisms can grow.

Hand cream Use a hand cream to keep your hands soft and supple. Avoid chapped hands. Cover cuts and abrasions with a clean waterproof plaster or sterile dressing to protect yourself from micro-organisms.

■ OSCE SCENARIO: INFECTION PREVENTION

Read the scenario and then perform the skill of hand-washing using the correct technique.

Mrs Susan Yates has been admitted to hospital with scabies and is in a side room. You have completed her care and now have to wash your hands before leaving the room.

- Hand-washing will be a component of every OSCE.
- Use the checklist below to practise the skill of hand-washing.

OSCE checklist: hand-washing assessment

SKILL	PERFORMED COMPETENTLY	PERFORMED BUT NOT COMPETENT	NOT PERFORMED/ INCOMPETENT
Communication – student informs the patient that he or she is going to wash their own hands			
Wets hands under running water and applies soap			
Washes hands using the Ayliffe procedure (eight steps)			

SKILL	PERFORMED COMPETENTLY	PERFORMED BUT NOT COMPETENT	NOT PERFORMED/ INCOMPETENT
Dries hands thoroughly using paper towels or other drying mechanism			
Pass/fail			

Scenarios for other branches of nursing

MENTAL HEALTH BRANCH

Mr James Burrows has been admitted to hospital with vomiting. He has also been complaining of stomach pains. You are the student nurse on duty and have been asked to get Mr Burrows a receiver and tissues. After caring for Mr Burrows, you need to wash your hands correctly.

CHILD AND YOUNG PERSON'S BRANCH

Veronica Tim is 5 years old and has been admitted with a flu virus to the children's ward. You are the student nurse on placement and have been asked to take care of Veronica. It is time for you to finish your shift and wash your hands before leaving.

LEARNING DISABILITY BRANCH

Mrs Tina Dunn is 22 years old and has learning disabilities. She has been admitted with a chest infection and head lice. You are a student nurse on the ward and have just treated the head lice. You now need to wash your hands.

Blood pressure measurement

■ EQUIPMENT REQUIRED TO MEASURE BLOOD PRESSURE

- Hand-rub
- Plastic apron
- Pillow
- Sphygmomanometer
- Stethoscope
- Wipes
- Observation chart
- Black pen

■ AIMS OF MEASURING BLOOD PRESSURE

- To establish a baseline observation (a reading to measure against).
- To detect deterioration or improvement of the patient's condition so that the appropriate action can be taken.
- To monitor the effects of prescribed medication, for example medication prescribed for high blood pressure (hypertension).

■ PROCEDURE OF MEASURING BLOOD PRESSURE

1. Wash your hands using the Ayliffe procedure.
2. Prepare the patient by introducing yourself and explain in simple terms what you are about to do.
3. Gain the patient's consent and gather the required equipment for the procedure (see above).
4. Place the correct-sized cuff 2–3 cm above the antecubital fossa, ensuring the centre of the inflatable

bladder is over the brachial artery (mid inner arm). Use the arrow on the cuff to guide you.

5. Estimate the systolic pressure to prevent the cuff being overinflated by feeling for the radial pulse, inflating the cuff until the radial pulse disappears under the fingertips and noting the measurement. Now deflate the cuff and wait 20 seconds for the arm to recover.

6. Inflate the cuff to 20–30 mmHg above the estimated systolic pressure.

7. Place the head of the stethoscope over the brachial artery at the antecubital fossa, pressing firmly. (This presses an artery over a bone, causing the bumping sound that you hear). Check that the drum of the stethoscope is working by tapping it gently whilst it is in your ears.

8. Listen for Korotkoff sounds as the cuff deflates and observe the reading. Control the gauge slowly.

9. Note the first (systolic) and last (diastolic) sounds only (you will hear swishing sounds in between – ignore these).

10. Deflate the cuff completely and remove the cuff from the arm.

11. Wash your hands using the Ayliffe procedure.

12. Record the reading on a clinical measurements chart and make the patient comfortable.

13. Inform a qualified nurse or doctor of any changes in the patient's condition.

■ TIPS TO SUCCESS IN YOUR OSCE

Communication skills Introduce yourself, saying your role and full name. Ask the patient's name and what they would like to be called.

Consent Always ask permission to proceed with the skill. You need to gain consent at all times.

Equipment Use only the equipment needed (see list above).

Infection prevention Always wash your hands using the Ayliffe procedure at the beginning and at the end of a procedure, and at any other times when necessary. Clean the ear pieces of the stethoscope after use (to prevent cross infection).

Privacy and dignity Be aware that the patient may have to remove some clothing so that you can apply the cuff. Ensure you maintain the patient's privacy and dignity at all times: close the curtains.

Results Blood pressure readings can alter with age and disease. An average blood pressure reading is 120/80 mmHg for an adult. Remember to look at baseline observations.

Position of patient, yourself and equipment while taking the blood pressure reading Ensure the patient is in a seated position with both feet on the floor, if possible. The chosen arm should be rested on a pillow on a flat surface. Do not use an arm where there may be a problem, for example where there is broken skin or an intravenous infusion. Do not ask the patient to hold their arm in place themselves as this may increase the blood pressure; instead, use a pillow to support the arm. Place the sphygmomanometer at heart level, on a steady surface next to the patient. Seat yourself at the patient's eye level to reassure them, as anxiety can affect the results. Always explain to the patient what you are doing, in terminology they will understand.

Positioning of cuff Ensure the appropriate size of cuff is used (small, medium, large or extra large). Cuffs that are too short or too large give inaccurate readings. Ensure that the patient's sleeves are rolled up comfortably to accommodate the cuff.

Estimated reading Find the radial pulse and inflate the cuff until the radial pulse disappears under your fingers. Note the measurement on the dial. Now deflate the cuff and wait 20 seconds before taking the final reading. This avoids the cuff inflating too much and causing discomfort for the patient.

Korotkoff sounds These are the two main sounds you are listening for when measuring blood pressure. Listen for the first sound coming in (systolic). Note this number. There will be swishing sounds in between. Listen for the last sound going out (diastolic). Note this number.

Documentation Ensure the blood pressure measurement is documented correctly using a black pen. The chart will vary in format according to where you are studying or working.

Report Report any abnormalities by comparing the patient's baseline observations with your results. Is the blood pressure lower or higher or the same?

Patient's comfort Always use a pillow to support the patient's arm while measuring the blood pressure. Ensure the patient is left in a comfortable position after the reading has been taken, and ask them if they require anything.

■ OSCE SCENARIO: MEASURING BLOOD PRESSURE

Read the scenario and then perform the skill of measuring blood pressure using the correct procedure. Remember that it is usual for the examiner to check the simulated patient's blood pressure at regular intervals during the OSCE.

Mrs Phyllis Jones is 70 years old and has a history of hypertension (high blood pressure). Mrs Jones has come to the GP clinic to have her blood pressure checked. You are the student nurse on clinical placement and have been asked by your mentor to perform the procedure of measuring blood pressure.

- Task to take 15 minutes – time yourself when practising.
- Perform the correct procedure of blood pressure on your patient.
- Use the checklist below to practise the skill of blood pressure measurement.

OSCE checklist: blood pressure measurement

SKILL	PERFORMED COMPETENTLY	PERFORMED BUT NOT COMPETENT	NOT PERFORMED/ INCOMPETENT
Communication – student introduces themselves and gains consent from patient			
Prepares patient and gathers equipment			
Washes hands using Ayliffe procedure			

SKILL	PERFORMED COMPETENTLY	PERFORMED BUT NOT COMPETENT	NOT PERFORMED/ INCOMPETENT
Positions sphygmomanometer at heart level			
Applies cuff 2–3 cm above the brachial pulse			
Estimates systolic blood pressure using radial pulse; deflates cuff			
Inflates cuff to estimated systolic reading plus 20–30 mmHg			
Measures blood pressure by defining systolic and diastolic readings			
Aftercare of patient – removes cuff and makes patient comfortable			
Washes hands using Ayliffe procedure			

SKILL	PERFORMED COMPETENTLY	PERFORMED BUT NOT COMPETENT	NOT PERFORMED/ INCOMPETENT
Documents results on an appropriate clinical measurements chart			
Overall approach to task			
Pass/fail			

Scenarios for other branches of nursing
MENTAL HEALTH BRANCH

Mr David Smith has been admitted to hospital with depression. He has also been complaining of headaches and dizziness. David has a history of hypotension (low blood pressure). You are the student nurse on clinical placement and have been asked by your mentor to perform the procedure of measuring blood pressure.

CHILD AND YOUNG PERSON'S BRANCH

Miss Lucy Car is 17 years old. She is visiting the GP practice nurse as she has been complaining of headaches and dizziness and has been stressed with examinations at school. You are the student nurse on clinical placement and have been asked by your mentor to perform the procedure of measuring blood pressure.

LEARNING DISABILITY BRANCH

Mrs Pauline Toms is 45 years old and has learning disabilities. She has recently been diagnosed with hypertension (high blood pressure). You are the student nurse on clinical placement and have been asked by your mentor to perform the procedure of measuring blood pressure.

Pulse and respiration measurement

■ EQUIPMENT REQUIRED TO MEASURE PULSE AND RESPIRATION

- Fob watch
- Observation chart
- Black pen

■ AIM OF MEASURING PULSE AND RESPIRATION

- To establish a baseline observation (a reading to measure against).
- To detect deterioration or improvement of a patient's condition so that the appropriate action can be taken.
- To monitor the effects of prescribed medication, for example to check whether an inhaler for the treatment of asthma has been effective.

■ PROCEDURE OF MEASURING PULSE AND RESPIRATION

1. Wash your hands using the Ayliffe procedure.
2. Reassure the patient and explain what you are about to do in simple terminology.
3. Gain the patient's consent to measure their pulse.

4. Locate the radial pulse in the wrist – place the pads of your second and third fingers in the hollow immediately above the wrist creases at the base of the thumb. Press lightly but sufficiently to feel the beats of the pulse.

5. Count the number of beats in a minute. Are the beats regular or irregular, weak or strong?

6. Continue to feel for the radial pulse and count the patient's respirations for a further minute. (Although you have gained consent at the beginning, it is helpful not to remind the patient you are counting the respirations, as this can alter the pattern of their breathing.)

7. Watch the patient's chest rise and fall (one respiration in and one respiration out is counted as one respiration).

8. Wash your hands using the Ayliffe procedure.

9. Record this reading on a clinical measurements chart and make the patient comfortable.

10. Inform a qualified nurse of any changes compared with the baseline observations.

■ OTHER OBSERVATIONS TO OBSERVE WHEN MEASURING RESPIRATION

- Are the respirations deep or shallow?
- Is there a cough present? If so, what type of cough? Is it tickly, dry or productive (producing sputum)?
- Is there a wheeze or a crackling sound? Any other sounds?
- What is the patient's general skin colour? Is it pink/pale/blue/white?
- Is there pain when breathing? How long does it last? What type of pain is it? How painful is the pain on a score of 1–10?

■ TIPS TO SUCCESS IN YOUR OSCE

Communication skills Introduce yourself, saying your role and full name. Ask the patient their name and what they would like to be called. **Remember**: this patient may be short of breath, so ask only closed questions.

Consent Always ask permission to proceed with the skill – you need to gain consent.

Equipment Use only the equipment needed (see list above).

Infection prevention Always wash your hands using the Ayliff procedure at the beginning and at the end of a procedure, and at other times when necessary.

Privacy and dignity Be aware that the patient may have to remove clothing so that you can access the radial pulse and see the chest rising and falling. Ensure you maintain the patient's privacy and dignity.

Results An average adult reading is 12–20 breaths a minute, but this may vary according to the patient's age and general condition.

Position of patient and yourself while timing the pulse and respirations Ensure the patient is in a comfortable position, preferably in an upright position. Seat yourself at the patient's eye level to reassure them, as anxiety can affect the results.

Timing Ensure the pulse and respirations are timed for a minute each. Notice the depth and rate of the beats. It may be a good idea to keep hold of the wrist while counting the respirations, as this takes the patient's mind off having their respirations counted. Try not to remind the patient that you are counting their respirations, as this may alter their breathing pattern.

Documentation Ensure that the pulse and respiration measurements are documented correctly using a black pen. The chart will vary in format according to where you are studying or working.

Report Report any abnormalities by comparing the result with the patient's baseline observations (observations taken on admission).

Patient's comfort Ensure the patient is left in a comfortable position after the procedure.

■ OSCE SCENARIO: MEASURING PULSE AND RESPIRATION

Read the scenario and then perform the skill of measuring pulse and respirations using the correct procedure. Remember that it is usual for the examiner to check the simulated patient's pulse and respirations at regular intervals during the OSCE.

Miss Jane Bennett is 30 years old. She has a history of a persistent cough and has been admitted with a mild asthma attack to the ward. You have been asked to measure Miss Bennett's pulse and respirations and then document them on the chart provided, reporting any results to a senior member of staff.

- Task to take 15 minutes – time yourself!
- Perform the measurement of pulse and respirations on your patient.
- Use the checklist below to practise the skill of pulse and respiration measurement.

OSCE checklist: pulse and respiration measurement

SKILL	PERFORMED COMPETENTLY	PERFORMED BUT NOT COMPETENT	NOT PERFORMED/ INCOMPETENT
Communication – student introduces themselves and gains consent from patient			
Prepares patient for procedure and gathers equipment			
Washes hands using Ayliffe procedure			
Locates radial pulse correctly			
Counts radial pulse for one minute			
Counts respirations for one minute			
Washes hands using the Ayliffe procedure			

SKILL	PERFORMED COMPETENTLY	PERFORMED BUT NOT COMPETENT	NOT PERFORMED/ INCOMPETENT
Documents the results correctly on clinical measurements chart provided			
Aftercare of patient – leaves patient comfortable			
Overall approach to task			
Pass/fail			

Scenarios for other branches of nursing
MENTAL HEALTH BRANCH

Mr Philip Smith has been admitted to hospital with anxiety. He has also been complaining of breathlessness and a cough. You are the student nurse on duty and have been asked to measure Mr Smith's pulse and respirations.

CHILD AND YOUNG PERSON'S BRANCH

Tim Kane is 14 years old. He is visiting the GP practice with his mother as he has recently had a chest infection. You are the student on placement and have been asked to measure his pulse and respirations.

LEARNING DISABILITY BRANCH

Mr Alan Gate is 23 years old and has learning disabilities. He has recently been diagnosed with bronchitis. You are a student nurse on the ward and have been asked by your mentor to measure his pulse and respirations.

Temperature measurement using a tympanic thermometer

■ EQUIPMENT REQUIRED TO MEASURE TEMPERATURE

- Observation chart
- Black pen
- Tympanic thermometer
- Tympanic thermometer covers

■ AIMS OF MEASURING TEMPERATURE

- To establish a baseline observation (a reading to measure against).
- To detect improvement or deterioration of a patient's condition.
- To monitor the effects of prescribed medication, for example paracetamol may be prescribed to reduce a patient's temperature.
- To monitor for signs of infection, for example a chest infection can produce a high temperature.
- To monitor for adverse affects when a patient has a blood transfusion.

■ PROCEDURE OF MEASURING TEMPERATURE

1. Wash your hands using the Ayliffe procedure.
2. Reassure the patient by introducing yourself and gain their consent.
3. Explain the procedure and equipment to be used in simple terms.
4. Ask the patient whether he or she has any problems with the ears, for example infection or past history of surgery.
5. Locate the tympanic aural mode in the window of the tympanic thermometer. Remember: there are two other modes – scan and timer – but these are not needed at this point.
6. Place a new cover on the tip of the probe (for infection prevention).
7. Place the probe into the ear canal so that it fits snugly (use a telephone position).
8. Press the scan button and wait to hear the continuous beeps.
9. Place the probe cover in a clinical waste bag using the eject button.
10. Wash your hands using the Ayliffe procedure.
11. Record the reading on the appropriate chart and make the patient comfortable.
12. Inform a qualified nurse of any changes to the patient's temperature.

■ TIPS TO SUCCESS IN YOUR OSCE

Communication skills Introduce yourself, stating your role and full name. Ask the patient their name and what they would like to be called.

Consent Always ask permission to proceed with the skill. You need to gain consent.

Equipment Use only the equipment needed (see list above).

Infection prevention Always wash your hands using the Ayliff procedure at the beginning and at the end of a procedure, and at other times when necessary.

Privacy and dignity Ensure you maintain the patient's privacy and dignity.

Position of patient and yourself while measuring the temperature Ensure the patient is in a seated position, with both feet on the floor. Seat yourself at the patient's eye level to reassure them, as anxiety can affect the results. Do not press the probe too firmly in the ear, as this may damage the ear; the probe should fit just snugly.

Timing The tympanic thermometer beeps when the temperature results are complete.

Documentation Ensure the temperature is documented correctly using a black pen. The chart will vary in format according to where you are studying or working.

Report Report any abnormalities by comparison with the patient's baseline observations.

Patient's comfort Ensure your patient is left in a comfortable position.

Observations Red-coloured skin may mean the patient
has a high temperature, which could indicate infection.
Pale skin may mean the patient is in shock. A blue
tinge may mean the patient has little oxygen circulating
around the body. Note if the patient is shivering or
sweating.

■ OSCE SCENARIO: MEASURING TEMPERATURE

Read the scenario and then perform the skill of measuring
a patient's temperature using the tympanic thermometer.
Remember it is usual for the examiner to check the simulated
patient's temperature at regular intervals.

Miss Isabel Jenkins is 33 years old and has been feeling
unwell. She has a history of a persistent cough and feeling
hot. You have been asked to measure Miss Jenkins'
temperature and then document the results on the chart
provided.

Remember: the tympanic mode must be selected in the
window before measuring the temperature. The other modes
are scan and timer.

- Task to take 15 minutes – time yourself.
- Perform the skill of measuring temperature using a
  tympanic thermometer.
- Use the checklist below to practise the skill of measuring
  a patient's temperature.

OSCE checklist: tympanic temperature measurement

SKILL	PERFORMED COMPETENTLY	PERFORMED BUT NOT COMPETENT	NOT PERFORMED/ INCOMPETENT
Communication: student introduces themselves and gains patient's consent			
Washes hands using Ayliffe procedure			
Selects tympanic mode on the screen			
Fits new probe cover			
Places probe tip in ear canal in correct position			
Presses and releases scan button			
Removes probe tip from ear when triple beeping sound goes off			

SKILL	PERFORMED COMPETENTLY	PERFORMED BUT NOT COMPETENT	NOT PERFORMED/ INCOMPETENT
Discards used probe cover in yellow bag using the eject button			
Reads temperature in window			
Washes hands using Ayliffe procedure			
Documents results on the chart provided			
Aftercare of patient			
Overall approach to task			
Pass/fail			

Scenarios for other branches of nursing

MENTAL HEALTH BRANCH

Mr Ronald Phipps has been admitted to hospital complaining of a fever and feeling unwell. Ronald has a history of chest infections. You are the student nurse on duty and have been asked to measure his temperature using a tympanic thermometer.

CHILD AND YOUNG PERSON'S BRANCH

David Gee is 7 year old and is visiting the GP practice with his mother. He has been complaining of fever symptoms. You are the student nurse on duty and have been asked to measure the temperature using a tympanic thermometer.

LEARNING DISABILITY BRANCH

Mr Sam Philips is 82 years old and has come into the emergency department with hypothermia. You are the student nurse on duty and have been asked to measure Mr Philips' temperature using a tympanic thermometer.

Aseptic technique

■ EQUIPMENT REQUIRED FOR ASEPTIC TECHNIQUE

- Apron
- Sterile dressing
- Dressing pack
- Gloves
- Tape
- Dressing trolley
- Cleaning solution

■ AIMS OF ASEPTIC TECHNIQUE

- To prevent the spread of infection.
- To promote wound healing.

■ PROCEDURE FOR ASEPTIC TECHNIQUE

1. Wash your hands using the Ayliffe procedure.
2. Reassure the patient, explain what you are about to do and gain the patient's consent.

3. In the clinical room, don an apron and gloves. Wash the aseptic trolley with soap and water and dry it (clean in one direction only). Then clean the trolley with cleaning wipes from top to bottom, (clean in one direction only). The top part of the trolley is the sterile field and must not be touched until the equipment is opened at the bedside.

4. Remove the apron and gloves (always apron first and then gloves) and discard into a clinical waste bag.

5. Wash your hands using the Ayliffe procedure.

6. Gather the equipment as above and display it on the bottom of the trolley. All equipment should be sterile, in date and unopened.

7. Take trolley to the patient's bedside, taking care not to touch the top of trolley, as this is the sterile field.

8. Wash your hands using the Ayliffe procedure.

9. Close the curtains for the patient's privacy and dignity.

10. Don an apron and gloves. Remove the used dressing and place it in a yellow bag.

11. Wash your hands using the Ayliffe procedure.

12. Open the dressing pack (check the expiry date on the packet) using the non-touch technique and empty it on to the trolley from a small height, so that the outside packaging does not touch the sterile field.

13. Open the cleaning solution, for example normal saline (check the expiry date on the packet). Pour into a gallipot from a small height so the outside packaging does not touch the sterile field.

14. Open the clean dressing (check the expiry date on the packet) on to the top of the trolley using the non-touch technique.

15. Place a sterile dressing sheet under the affected area, using non-touch. Ask the patient to lift up the affected area (for example, the arm) so that you can slide the sheet underneath.
16. Don the correct size of sterile gloves, as instructed.
17. Clean the wound as instructed, using the one-way system.
18. Dry the wound as instructed, using the one-way system.
19. Place a clean dressing on the wound and secure it.
20. Dispose of waste, apron and gloves into the yellow bag provided and seal. Leave the sealed bag on top of the trolley.
21. Wash your hands using the Ayliffe procedure.
22. Ensure the patient is comfortable.
23. Dispose of clinical waste in sluice.
24. Clean the trolley before returning it to the treatment area.
25. Document the following: time of dressing, colour of wound, depth of wound, smell of wound, any improvement?, dressing used, size of wound.

■ TIPS TO SUCCESS IN YOUR OSCE

Communication skills Introduce yourself, stating your role and full name. Ask the patient their name and what they would like to be called.

Consent Always ask permission to proceed with the skill. You need to gain consent.

Equipment Use only the equipment needed (see list above). Check in the patient's notes to see what dressing is required.

Infection prevention Always wash your hands using the Ayliffe procedure at the beginning and at the end of a procedure, and at other times when necessary.

Privacy and dignity Be aware that the patient may not want to look at their wound and may be embarrassed for others to see it. Ensure the curtains are drawn to maintain the patient's privacy and dignity.

Position of patient and yourself while changing the dressing Ensure the patient is in a comfortable position, with the affected area supported. Seat yourself at the patient's level to avoid stooping.

Timing Ask the patient if they would like to use the toilet before you start the procedure and after the dressing change is complete.

Documentation Ensure the wound documentation is correct and written in black pen.

Report Report any changes to the nurse in charge.

Patient's comfort Offer pain relief as prescribed before performing the wound dressing. Ensure the patient is in a comfortable position during and after the procedure.

■ OSCE SCENARIO: ASEPTIC TECHNIQUE

Read the scenario and then perform the skill of aseptic technique.

Mrs Paula Lamb has arrived at the accident and emergency department with a laceration to her right leg after a fall. You have been asked to set up a trolley in preparation for cleaning and dressing the wound. Once you have set up the dressing trolley, perform the aseptic technique on Mrs Lamb's wound.

- Task to take 15 minutes – time yourself!
- Perform the procedure of the aseptic technique on your patient.
- Use the checklist below to practise the skill of the aseptic technique.

OSCE checklist: changing a wound dressing using the aseptic technique

SKILL	PERFORMED COMPETENTLY	PERFORMED BUT NOT COMPETENT	NOT PERFORMED/ INCOMPETENT
Communication: student introduces themselves to patient and gains patient's consent			
Washes hands using Ayliffe procedure			
Dons apron and gloves			
Cleans and dries trolley			
Gathers correct equipment and places on bottom shelf of trolley			
Prepares patient for procedure with privacy and dignity maintained			
Washes hands using Ayliffe technique			

SKILL	PERFORMED COMPETENTLY	PERFORMED BUT NOT COMPETENT	NOT PERFORMED/ INCOMPETENT
Dons apron and gloves			
Removes dressing using non-touch technique and places dressing in a yellow bag			
Removes apron and gloves into clinical waste bag			
Washes hands using Ayliffe procedure			
Dons apron and gloves			
Opens dressing pack and other equipment on to trolley, avoiding contamination and checking expiry dates			
Applies sterile gloves, avoiding contamination			

SKILL	PERFORMED COMPETENTLY	PERFORMED BUT NOT COMPETENT	NOT PERFORMED/ INCOMPETENT
Uses aseptic technique to clean round the wound and dry the wound			
Applies clean dressing			
Disposes of equipment in yellow bag			
Aftercare of patient			
Overall approach to task			
Pass/fail			

Scenarios for other branches of nursing

MENTAL HEALTH BRANCH

Mr Layton Smith has been admitted to hospital with suicidal tendencies. Mr Smith has attempted to cut his wrists and has caused trauma to his right wrist. You are the student nurse on duty and have been asked to clean the wound using the aseptic technique.

CHILD AND YOUNG PERSON'S BRANCH

Tina Dodd is 8 years old and is visiting the GP practice nurse after sustaining a cut to her hand from a fall. You are the student nurse on placement and have been asked to perform a wound dressing on her hand using the aseptic technique.

LEARNING DISABILITY BRANCH

Tom Dillon is 16 years old and has learning disabilities. He has recently had an operation on his abdomen, which has left him with a wound. You are the student nurse on placement and have been asked to perform a wound dressing on the abdomen using the aseptic technique.

Elimination needs: stool specimen

■ EQUIPMENT REQUIRED TO COLLECT A STOOL SPECIMEN

- Apron
- Gloves
- Specimen bag and request form
- Black pen
- Stool collection container
- Bed pan and cover

■ AIMS OF COLLECTING A STOOL SPECIMEN

- To maintain infection-prevention measures.
- To obtain a sample of faeces using the appropriate equipment.
- To send a stool specimen to the laboratory.

■ PROCEDURE FOR STOOL COLLECTION

1. Explain to the patient the reason for the collection of the stool specimen and the test required. Ensure that the bed pan is labelled with the patient's name.

2. Wash your hands using the Ayliffe procedure.
3. Don gloves and an apron. (Wear gloves and an apron when handling any bodily fluids.)
4. Obtain a stool specimen from the patient and take the specimen to the sluice.
5. Use the spoon/scoop attached to the lid of the specimen container to transfer a portion of the faeces to the specimen container. Do not touch the specimen, because it is contaminated.
6. Discard the remaining faeces appropriately.
7. Discard the gloves and apron.
8. Wash your hands using the Ayliffe procedure.
9. Label the specimen container with the patient's details. Complete the appropriate laboratory request form, noting any special instructions ordered by the doctor.

■ TIPS TO SUCCESS IN YOUR OSCE

Communication skills Introduce yourself, stating your role and full name. Ask the patient their name and what they would like to be called.

Consent Gain the patient's consent to send a stool specimen to the laboratory.

Equipment Use only the equipment needed (see list above).

Infection prevention Always wash your hands using the Ayliffe procedure at the beginning and at the end of a procedure, and at other times when necessary.

Privacy and dignity When the patient is providing the specimen, ensure they have privacy and dignity.

Correct specimen container Ensure the appropriate specimen container is used, with a spoon or a scoop attached to the lid.

Observation of stool specimen Compare the faeces against the Bristol stool chart (see below) and document in the patient's nursing notes.

Bristol stool chart

Type 1		Separate hard lumps, like nuts (hard to pass)
Type 2		Sausage-shaped but lumpy
Type 3		Like a sausage but with cracks on its surface
Type 4		Like a sausage or snake, smooth and soft
Type 5		Soft blobs with clear-cut edges (passed easily)
Type 6		Fluffy pieces with ragged edges, a mushy stool
Type 7		Watery, no solid pieces **Entirely liquid**

From Lewis SJ, Heaton KW (1997) Stool form scale as a useful guide to intestinal transit time. *Scandinavian Journal of Gastroenterology* **32**(9):920–24. © Informa Healthcare

Documentation Ensure the procedure of stool collection for a specimen is documented correctly using a black pen. The patient may be on a stool chart. The chart will vary in format according to where you are studying or working.

Report Report any abnormalities.

Patient comfort Ensure the patient is left in a comfortable position and ask them if they require anything.

■ OSCE SCENARIO: COLLECTING A STOOL SPECIMEN

Read the scenario and then perform the skill of stool collection using the correct procedure.

Mr Paul Dillon is 40 years old and has a history of constipation. Mr Dillon has come into hospital for investigations. The doctor has requested that Mr Dillon provides a stool specimen for testing in the laboratory. You are the student nurse on duty. Perform the skill of stool collection.

- Task to take 15 minutes – time yourself!
- Perform the procedure of stool collection.
- Use the checklist below to practise the skill of stool collection.

OSCE checklist: stool collection

SKILL	PERFORMED COMPETENTLY	PERFORMED BUT NOT COMPETENT	NOT PERFORMED/ INCOMPETENT
Communication: student introduces themselves and gains consent from patient			
Student prepares patient and gathers equipment			

SKILL	PERFORMED COMPETENTLY	PERFORMED BUT NOT COMPETENT	NOT PERFORMED/ INCOMPETENT
Washes hands using Ayliffe procedure			
Dons apron and gloves			
Uses scoop or spoon to collect stool sample			
Places sample in pot and closes lid			
Discards bed pan contents appropriately			
Places apron and gloves in clinical waste bag			
Washes hands using Ayliffe procedure			
Ensures patient is comfortable			
Fills in label on the specimen container			

SKILL	PERFORMED COMPETENTLY	PERFORMED BUT NOT COMPETENT	NOT PERFORMED/ INCOMPETENT
Places specimen in plastic bag with the request form to be sent to the laboratory			
Overall approach to task			
Pass/fail			

Scenarios for other branches of nursing

MENTAL HEALTH BRANCH

Mrs Ann Price has been admitted to hospital with anorexia. She has been complaining of stomach cramps and blood in her stool. You are the student nurse admitting this patient. Ask the patient for a stool specimen and collect a stool specimen for the laboratory.

CHILD AND YOUNG PERSON'S BRANCH

Bert Woods is 5 years old and has been admitted with constipation. You are the student nurse admitting this child. Collect a stool specimen for the laboratory.

LEARNING DISABILITY BRANCH

Mr Adam Nun is 22 years old and is immobile in a wheelchair. He has stomach pain and vomiting. You are the student nurse on duty. Collect a stool specimen for the laboratory.

Elimination needs: urine testing (urinalysis)

■ **EQUIPMENT REQUIRED TO TEST URINE**

- Gloves
- Plastic apron
- Fob watch
- Urinalysis testing strips
- Black pen
- Paper towel
- Yellow waste bag
- Urinalysis results chart

■ **AIM OF COLLECTING AND TESTING URINE**

- To detect changes in a patient's condition through testing urine with urine testing strips.

Normal urine is straw-coloured and clear. If the urine looks cloudy or contains debris, it may indicate infection or disease. If the urine has an odour, for example a fishy smell, it may indicate infected urine.

■ **PROCEDURE FOR TESTING URINE**

1. Wash your hands using the Ayliffe procedure.
2. Prepare the patient by explaining the procedure and gain their consent.
3. Gather the required equipment (as above).
4. Ask the patient to provide a specimen of urine in a clean container.
5. Take the specimen of urine to the sluice.
6. Wash your hands using the Ayliffe procedure.
7. Don an apron and gloves.

8. Check the date on the testing strips, remove one strip from the container and close the lid tightly. Check the expiry date on the container.

9. Dip the stick into the urine, ensuring all pads are covered with urine. Take the strip straight out of the urine, wiping the pads against the side to remove excess urine (always check the individual instructions on the container).

10. Place the testing strip on a clean paper towel, the correct way up, next to the testing strip container (ensure that you can see the diagram that shows you what the results mean).

11. Time the test for one minute (or as directed on the testing strip container).

12. While the urinalysis stick is being timed, take off the apron and gloves and wash your hands.

13. After one minute, note the results against the chart provided without touching the urine stick or the container.

14. Don an apron and gloves and dispose of the testing stick and paper towel in the clinical waste bag. Take off the apron and gloves and dispose of them in a clinical waste bag.

15. Wash your hands using the Ayliffe procedure.

■ TIPS TO SUCCESS IN YOUR OSCE

Communication skills Introduce yourself, giving your role and full name. Ask the patient their name and what they would like to be called.

Consent Always ask permission to proceed with the urinalysis test.

Equipment Use only the equipment needed (see list above).

Infection prevention Always wash your hands using the Ayliffe procedure at the beginning and at the end of a procedure, and at other times where necessary. Do not let the testing strip touch the side of the testing strip container or your pen, as this will cause contamination.

Privacy and dignity Be aware that the patient will have to provide a fresh specimen of urine before you test the urine. Do not test the urine in front of the patient.

Positioning of testing strip Ensure the testing strip is the correct way up when reading the results. Line up the testing strip with the side of the testing strip container that shows the results.

Documentation Ensure each result is correctly documented and signed for. When checking the results, compare the correct urine pad with the correct-coloured square on the chart provided.

Report Report any abnormalities to a trained nurse.

■ OSCE SCENARIO: URINE TESTING

Read the scenario and then perform the skill of testing urine using the correct procedure.

Mrs Denise Blade is 47 years old and has a history of urinary tract infections. She has come to the GP clinic to have her urine tested. You are the student nurse on duty and have been asked by your mentor to test Mrs Blade's urine using the urine testing sticks provided.

- Task to take 15 minutes – time yourself!
- Perform the procedure of testing urine.
- Use the checklist below to practise the skill of urinalysis.

OSCE checklist: urinalysis

SKILL	PERFORMED COMPETENTLY	PERFORMED BUT NOT COMPETENT	NOT PERFORMED/ INCOMPETENT
Communication: student introduces themselves and gains patient's consent; collects specimen			
Washes hands using Ayliffe procedure			
Dons aprons and gloves			
Removes reagent strip from container, after checking expiry date			
Dips the reagent strip in the urine and withdraws the strip immediately, tapping the side on the container			

SKILL	PERFORMED COMPETENTLY	PERFORMED BUT NOT COMPETENT	NOT PERFORMED/ INCOMPETENT
Times the urine test for 60 seconds before reading the results; takes off gloves and apron and washes hands			
Reads the test strip against the chart on the container, ensuring the strip does not touch the side of the container			
Records the results on the urinalysis chart			
Dons apron and gloves			
Disposes of reagent strip and urine correctly			

SKILL	PERFORMED COMPETENTLY	PERFORMED BUT NOT COMPETENT	NOT PERFORMED/ INCOMPETENT
Washes hands using Ayliffe procedure			
Overall approach to the task	＇		
Pass/fail			

Scenarios for other branches of nursing

MENTAL HEALTH BRANCH

Mr Timothy Taylor is 74 years old has been admitted to hospital with depression. He has not been bathing at home and has been complaining of symptoms of a urinary tract infection. You are the student nurse on duty and have been asked to admit Mr Taylor and test his urine routinely.

CHILD AND YOUNG PERSON'S BRANCH

Miss Amanda Riley is 17 years old and has come into hospital with unstable diabetes. You are the student nurse on placement and have been asked to test Miss Riley's urine.

LEARNING DISABILITY BRANCH

Mr Don Samson is 26 years old and has a suprapubic catheter. He has recently complained of cloudy urine. You have been asked to test his urine.

Intramuscular injection technique

■ EQUIPMENT REQUIRED TO ADMINISTER AN INTRAMUSCULAR INJECTION

- Apron
- Gloves
- Black pen
- Prescription sheet
- Sharps box
- Swab
- Gauze
- Syringes × 2
- Needles (use the appropriate size for the patient)
- Injection tray
- Medication as prescribed

■ AIM OF ADMINISTERING AN INTRAMUSCULAR INJECTION

- To safely administer prescribed medication using an intramuscular injection.

■ PROCEDURE FOR INTRAMUSCULAR INJECTION TECHNIQUE USING THE DORSOGLUTEAL REGION (UPPER OUTER QUADRANT OF THE BUTTOCK)

In the OSCE the examiner may be the second checker (qualified nurse). As a student, in clinical practice you would only be allowed to observe a drug round.

1. Explain to the patient the reason for administering an injection and gain their consent.

2. Check for any special requirements and allergies.
3. Wash your hands using the Ayliffe procedure.
4. Check the prescription sheet, medication and equipment required with the trained nurse. Check on the prescription sheet that the following are documented: route (IM, intramuscular), correct site, amount of medication prescribed, doctor's signature, date prescribed, time injection due.
5. **Remember**: if any of these items is missing from the prescription sheet, the injection cannot be given until the prescription sheet has been rectified.
6. Select the correct size of needle and syringe to draw up the medication as prescribed.
7. Draw up the correct amount of medication using the correct size of syringe and needle. Check all air bubbles are removed from the solution.
8. Change the needle for the administration of the medication. **DO NOT RESHEATH** a needle under any circumstances, to avoid needle-stick injury.
9. Wash your hands using the Ayliffe procedure.
10. Take the drawn-up medication and swab on a medication tray with the prescription sheet and sharps box to the patient's bedside.
11. Check against the prescription sheet that you have:
    - the correct patient;
    - the correct hospital number;
    - the correct prescribed medication;
    - the correct route;
    - the correct injection site;
    - the doctor's signature and date prescribed.

12. Draw the curtains to maintain the patient's privacy and dignity. Keep the patient's body covered as much as possible.
13. Wash your hands using the Ayliffe procedure.
14. Ask the patient to lie or stand in the appropriate position, according to the injection site to be used. Check the prescription sheet and medication vial again with the trained nurse.
15. Check again that you have the right patient with a trained nurse (in the OSCE, the examiner may offer to be the second checker).
16. A popular injection site is the dorsogluteal region (upper outer quadrant of buttock); use an imaginary cross to outline the area.

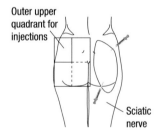

Outer upper quadrant for injections

Sciatic nerve

17. Swab the site in one direction only and wait for it to dry.
18. Stretch the skin and inject at 90 degrees, leaving a quarter of the needle out of the skin.
19. Pull back on the plunger (only slightly, to avoid too much air entering the syringe). If no blood appears in the barrel

of the syringe, continue to inject slowly, talking to your
patient to reassure them.
20. Pull the needle out and then let go of the skin.
21. Put the syringe and needle in the sharps box.
22. Wash your hands using the Ayliffe procedure.
23. The trained nurse should sign for the injection on the
prescription sheet.
24. After the injection, revisit the patient to assess the
injected site for any allergic reactions or side effects
from the medication, for example a rash or redness.
Report your findings to a trained nurse.

■ TIPS TO SUCCESS IN YOUR OSCE

Communication skills Introduce yourself, stating your role
and full name. Ask the patient their name and what they
would like to be called.

Consent Always ask permission to proceed with
administrating an injection.

Equipment Use only the equipment needed (see list above).

Infection prevention Always wash your hands using the
Ayliffe procedure at the beginning and at the end of a
procedure, and at other times when necessary.

Privacy and dignity When the patient is in the correct position
for you to administer the prescribed medication, ensure their
privacy and dignity are maintained at all times, for example
the curtains drawn and the patient covered with a sheet.

Correct size of syringe and needle Ensure the appropriate
size of syringe and needle are used to administer
medication by intramuscular injection. Each patient should
be assessed individually according to their size, build and
weight.

Correct positioning and site Ensure the patient is the correct position before administering the prescribed medication. Use alternate sites to avoid bruising, breakdown of skin and abscesses. Avoid injecting sites with broken skin.

Documentation Ensure the procedure of the injection technique is documented correctly, stating the site used, route, medication prescribed and any problems that occur during the procedure. Use a diagram to show where the injection was given last.

Report Report any abnormalities or side effects that occur after administration of the medication.

Patient's comfort Ensure the patient is left in a comfortable position after the administration of the medication.

■ OSCE SCENARIO: INTRAMUSCULAR INJECTION TECHNIQUE

Read the scenario and then perform the skill of administrating medication via a intramuscular injection. In an OSCE a manikin will be used for the injection procedure.

Mr David Man is 60 years old and has been diagnosed with terminal cancer. To control Mr Man's pain, he has been prescribed an injection of diamorphine. Your mentor will watch you check/draw up the medication as prescribed, and then you should demonstrate giving an intramuscular injection on the manikin.

- Task to take 15 minutes – time yourself!
- Perform the procedure of intramuscular injection on the manikin.
- Use the checklist below to practise the skill of intramuscular injection technique.

OSCE checklist: intramuscular injection technique

SKILL	PERFORMED COMPETENTLY	PERFORMED BUT NOT COMPETENT	NOT PERFORMED/ INCOMPETENT
Communication: student introduces themselves and gains patient's consent			
Washes hands using Ayliffe procedure			
Dons gloves			
Verbally examines drug chart for vital information against drug vial			
Selects and prepares correct equipment and draws up drug correctly			
Identifies the correct patient, checking against the prescription sheet and patient's arm band			

SKILL	PERFORMED COMPETENTLY	PERFORMED BUT NOT COMPETENT	NOT PERFORMED/ INCOMPETENT
Positions patient and identifies choice of Injection site			
Performs intramuscular injection using correct technique			
Disposes of waste in sharps box			
Washes hands using Ayliffe procedure			
Signs prescription sheet with trained nurse			
Overall approach to task			
Pass/fail			

Scenarios for other branches of nursing
MENTAL HEALTH BRANCH
Miss Samantha Holland is 22 years old and has been admitted to hospital with depression after the death of her mother. Miss Holland is due her intramuscular injection and you are the student nurse on duty.

Your mentor will watch you check and draw up the medication as prescribed and demonstrate giving an intramuscular injection on a manikin.

CHILD AND YOUNG PERSON'S BRANCH
Charlie Sand is 10 years old and has recently arrived back on the ward after having a major operation. Charlie has woken up feeling sick and in pain and needs an injection as prescribed for the sickness. Your mentor will watch you check and draw up the medication as prescribed and demonstrate giving an intramuscular injection on a manikin.

LEARNING DISABILITY BRANCH
Miss Cynthia Ray is 32 years old and has come to the GP with her carer for a tetanus injection. Your mentor will watch you check and draw up the medication as prescribed and demonstrate giving an intramuscular injection on a manikin.

Administering oral fluids and fluid balance

■ EQUIPMENT REQUIRED TO ADMINISTER MEASURED ORAL FLUIDS

- Measuring container
- Cup or glass
- Tissues
- Fluids, for example water
- Black pen
- Fluid balance chart

■ AIMS OF ADMINISTERING ORAL FLUIDS

- To maintain hydration of the patient.
- To observe and record patient's intake and output of fluids.

- To maintain fluid balance chart.
- To detect deterioration and improvement of patient's condition.

■ PROCEDURE OF ADMINISTERING ORAL FLUIDS

1. Wash your hands using the Ayliffe procedure.
2. Prepare the patient, gain their consent and gather equipment as above.
3. Ensure the patient is sitting upright to maintain digestion.
4. Check the patient's fluid balance chart to identify the required amount of fluid and the correct time to administer the fluid to the patient.
5. Measure the required amount of fluid into a measuring container.
6. Ensure the container is placed flat on a surface before pouring out the required amount, to ensure accuracy.
7. Give the fluid to the patient, helping them as required.
8. Offer a tissue to wipe the mouth and dispose of it in a clinical waste bag.
9. Document the amount of fluid administered on the fluid balance chart and in the patient's notes.
10. Dispose of the drinking vessel accordingly.
11. Ensure the patient is comfortable.
12. Wash your hands using the Ayliffe procedure.
13. Inform a qualified nurse of any changes in the patient's condition.

■ TIPS TO SUCCESS IN YOUR OSCE

Communication skills Introduce yourself, stating your role and full name. Ask the patient their name and what they would like to be called.

Consent Always ask permission to proceed with the procedure.

Equipment Use only the equipment needed (see list above).

Infection prevention Always wash your hands using the Ayliffe procedure at the beginning and at the end of a procedure, and at other times when necessary.

Privacy and dignity Be aware that the patient may have underlying medical problems, for example dribbling caused by a cerebral vascular accident (stroke). Maintain the patient's privacy and dignity.

Positioning of patient Ensure the patient is sat upright so that normal digestion of fluid takes place.

Documentation Ensure each time fluid is administered to the patient the amount is documented on the fluid balance chart and in the patient's notes.

Report Report any concerns to a qualified nurse, for example if the patient has problems with swallowing.

Patient's comfort After the procedure, check the patient is left in a comfortable position.

■ OSCE SCENARIO: ADMINISTERING ORAL FLUIDS

Miss Ann Wells is 65 years old and has undergone a surgical procedure. Miss Wells has returned to the ward and is able to have 10 ml of water every hour on the hour, on instructions from the doctor. It is 2p.m. and Miss Wells is due her 10 ml of water. Administer and document the fluid correctly.

- Task to take 15 minutes – time yourself!
- Perform the procedure of administering oral fluids to your patient.
- Use the checklist below to practise the skill of administering fluids to your patient.

OSCE checklist: administrating oral fluids

SKILL	PERFORMED COMPETENTLY	PERFORMED BUT NOT COMPETENT	NOT PERFORMED/ INCOMPETENT
Communication: student introduces themselves and gains patient's consent			
Determines how much water needs to be given to the patient by reading the patient's notes			
Washes hands using Ayliffe procedure			
Checks fluid balance chart to ascertain amount of fluid required; measures appropriate amount of water in measuring container			

SKILL	PERFORMED COMPETENTLY	PERFORMED BUT NOT COMPETENT	NOT PERFORMED/ INCOMPETENT
Positions patient in an upright position			
Offers a tissue for any spillage			
Asks patient to drink required amount of water			
On completion, ensures patient is comfortable; disposes of tissue			
Washes hands using Ayliffe procedure			
Records amount of fluid taken by the patient on the fluid balance chart			
Ensures the patient is comfortable			
Pass/fail			

Scenarios for other branches of nursing

MENTAL HEALTH BRANCH

Mr Ronald Baker is 87 years old and has been admitted to hospital with dehydration. He has not been drinking fluids at home. You are the student nurse on duty and have been asked to administer 20 ml of fluid to Mr Baker every hour, on the hour, and record it on his fluid balance chart.

CHILD AND YOUNG PERSON'S BRANCH

Miss Samantha Jones is 7 years old and has come into hospital with urinary tract infection. You are the student nurse on placement and have been asked to encourage fluids and offer 20 ml hourly. Document the fluid taken every hour on the fluid balance chart.

LEARNING DISABILITY BRANCH

Mr Donald Vickers is 56 years old and has returned from theatre. After 8 hours you are instructed by the doctor to give 10 ml fluid hourly until otherwise instructed and to document on the fluid balance chart provided.

Cardiopulmonary resuscitation (CPR)

■ EQUIPMENT REQUIRED TO ADMINISTER CPR

- Wipes or pocket mask

■ AIMS OF ADMINISTERING CPR

- To massage the heart and ventilate the lungs until the emergency services arrive or until the patient's heart restarts.
- To maintain the patient's airway, breathing and circulation.

■ PROCEDURE FOR ADMINISTERING CPR

1. **Initial assessment of the area** On approaching the casualty, always check for danger, such as traffic, water or electricity. Protect yourself – two casualties are no good to anyone! Check the person is not attached to electricity; if they are, switch off the mains before attending to them.
2. Kneel down by the person, shake them and shout in their ear 'Hello, can you hear me?'
3. If there is no response and no sign of life, shout for help. **If you are on your own with no one in sight, go and seek help first. Use the nearest phone.**
4. **Airway** Check in the person's mouth for any form of obstruction. Do not try to remove the obstruction, in case you push the object in further, unless the object is visibly removable without harming the patient.
5. **Breathing** Open the person's airway by placing one hand on the forehead and two fingers of the other hand under the chin and tilt the head back.

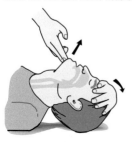

6. Place your cheek against the person's cheek, looking down their chest for 10 seconds and counting aloud. Look for the chest rising, listen for breaths, and feel for breath on your cheek.
7. **If there are still no signs of life**, shout for help and ask for an automated external defibrillator (AED) if one is available.
8. Perform cardiac compressions (30 compressions) by placing the heel of your hand on the centre of the sternum, in line with the nipples. Your arms should be kept straight, with your body leaning slightly over the person's chest.
9. Press down 5–6 cm on the chest and count the compressions out loud (Rate: 100–120 per minute).
10. After 30 compressions, give two breaths by opening the airway (place one hand on the forehead and two fingers under the chin and tilt the chin back) and placing your mouth over the causality's mouth; create a good seal between your mouth and the casualty's mouth. Pinch the nose at the same time.
11. Do not discontinue CPR unless the casualty starts to show signs of life.
12. Continue with this sequence of 30 compressions and 2 breaths until the casualty's heart starts, the emergency team arrives or you are too tired to continue.
13. **Shout for help again if no help has arrived.**
14. If the casualty starts breathing and has a cardiac output, a top-to-toe assessment should be carried out. The casualty should then be placed in the recovery

position (unless there are complications) until emergency help arrives.

15. Remember to note all events so that you can give an accurate report to the emergency services when they arrive.

■ TIPS TO SUCCESS IN YOUR OSCE

Communication skills Call for emergency help so that the casualty can be transferred to hospital as soon as possible. When telephoning the emergency services, state your name, the person's condition, sex and age, and the address of the event. Kneel down and shake and shout in the casualty's ear to ascertain whether they are conscious or not.

Equipment Use only the equipment needed and if available (see list above).

Infection prevention Always wash your hands at the end of a procedure using the Ayliffe procedure.

Privacy and dignity Be aware that the casualty's body may be exposed due to the procedure of chest compressions. Maintain their privacy and dignity as much as possible. Clothing may have to be removed to reach the chest area.

Position of casualty and yourself whilst performing CPR Ensure the person is laid flat. Ensure your hands are correctly positioned in the centre of the sternum (in line with the nipples), and your arms are kept straight. If the person returns to consciousness, put them in the recovery position, keeping the airway open.

Mouth-to-mouth When performing artificial respiration, ensure your mouth has a good seal over the casualty's mouth to prevent air escaping. Use a pocket mask if available.

CPR ratio 30 compressions to 2 breaths. The compressions should be 5–6 cm in depth (Rate: 100–120 per minute).

Recovery position This is the position that the casualty is placed in once they regain consciousness. Maintain observation at all times while the patient is in your care.

Documentation Ensure all events are reported to the emergency services.

■ OSCE SCENARIO: ADMINISTERING CPR

Read the scenario and then perform the skill of CPR using the correct procedure.

Mr Horace Wedge is 60 years old and has a history of angina and high blood pressure (hypertension). He has come to the accident and emergency department with chest pain. Mr Wedge suddenly collapses, with no signs of life. You are the student nurse on duty. Assess the situation and perform CPR until you are told to stop.

- Task to take 15 minutes – time yourself!
- Use the checklist below to practise the skill of CPR on the manikin provided.

OSCE checklist: administering CPR

SKILL	PERFORMED COMPETENTLY	PERFORMED BUT NOT COMPETENT	NOT PERFORMED/ INCOMPETENT
Checks environment for any danger			
Establishes casualty's unresponsiveness: shake and shout 'Hello! Can you hear me?'			
Shouts for help			
Looks in casualty's mouth for any obstructions			
Effectively opens airway using head-tilt or chin-lift			
Establishes apnoea by looking for the chest rising, listening for breath sounds and feeling for breath on cheek for 10 seconds			
Shouts for an automated external defibrillator			

SKILL	PERFORMED COMPETENTLY	PERFORMED BUT NOT COMPETENT	NOT PERFORMED/ INCOMPETENT
Correctly positions hands – middle of sternum, using heel of hands only			
Positions shoulders above sternum, with arms straight			
Depresses sternum 5–6 cm per compression			
Opens airway, pinches nose and breathes twice into person via mouth			
Checks that ventilation is adequate (chest should rise)			
Performs CPR at a rate of 30 compressions : two breaths			
Continues CPR until examiner instructs to stop			
Pass/fail			

Scenarios for other branches of nursing

MENTAL HEALTH BRANCH

Miss Susan Hodges has been admitted to hospital with depression. She has a history of attempting suicide. You are the student nurse on duty and have found Miss Hodges collapsed on the ground, with an empty bottle of tablets in her hand. There are no signs of life. Assess the situation and perform the correct procedure for CPR.

CHILD AND YOUNG PERSON'S BRANCH

Karl Grahame is 16 years old and has severe asthma. You are the student nurse in a community placement and have found Karl collapsed on the floor in the kitchen. There are no signs of life. Assess the situation and perform the correct procedure for CPR.

LEARNING DISABILITY BRANCH

Mrs Vera Acorn is known to have epilepsy. After she has a seizure in the street, you find her collapsed. There are no signs of life. Assess the situation and perform the correct procedure for CPR.

Oral drug administration

Please remember that only a trained nurse can administer prescribed medication. If a controlled drug is to be given, two trained nurses should check the prescription sheet.

■ EQUIPMENT REQUIRED TO ADMINISTER DRUGS ON A MEDICATION ROUND

- Hand-rub
- Prescription sheet

- Medicine pot
- Medicine tray
- Drug cart
- Medication
- Black pen
- Fob watch
- Gloves

■ AIMS OF DRUG ADMINISTRATION

- To safely administer prescribed medication to the patient.

■ PROCEDURE OF DRUG ADMINISTRATION

A trained nurse needs to check drug administration – ask the examiner to be the second checker.

1. Wash your hands using the Ayliffe procedure.
2. Prepare the patient, gain their consent and gather equipment as above.
3. Check the prescription sheet against the medication prescribed.
4. Check the name of the drug. Most drugs have two names – the generic name and the manufacturer's name. If you are unsure what the medication is used for, check with the local pharmacy or in the *British National Formulary* (BNF).
5. Check the patient's identification. Check their name against the prescription sheet and the patient's arm band. If the patient has not got an arm band, one must be issued before any drugs are administered.
6. Check the correct dose has been prescribed. Use the BNF to check the dose.

7. Check the route by which the medication is to be administered, for example intramuscular (IM) injection.

8. Check the time the medication should be given. Check how often the medication is to be given and when the last dose was given.

9. The doctor who completed the prescription sheet should have signed the correct signature box.

10. Check the prescription sheet for any allergies the patient may have.

11. Check any extra instructions, for example some prescriptions state 'give with food'. Clinical observations may need to be taken before administration of medication.

12. A trained nurse should sign for the administration of medication. In the case of controlled drugs, two trained nurses should sign the prescription sheet and controlled drug book.

13. If a cream is prescribed, the nurse should wear gloves to administer it, as some creams may aggravate the skin or have a thinning affect, for example steroids.

14. **If any of the above points are not in place or are incorrect, the medication must not be given.**

15. Use a clean medicine pot for each patient.

16. Do not mix tablets and liquids in the same pot.

17. If tablets need to be crushed, use a pestle and mortar. Tablets should be broken in half only if they are scored through the middle.

18. Offer the patient water to help them swallow the medication.

19. Wash your hands using the Ayliffe procedure.

20. Record the medication in the patient's prescription sheet and case notes.
21. Discard any equipment appropriately.
22. Chain the trolley back to the wall and lock it.

■ TIPS TO SUCCESS IN YOUR OSCE

Communication skills Introduce yourself, giving your role and full name. Ask the patient their name and what they would like to be called.

Consent Always ask the patient's permission to proceed with the drug administration.

Equipment Use only the equipment needed (see list above).

Infection prevention Always wash your hands using the Ayliffe procedure at the beginning and at the end of a procedure, and at other times when necessary.

Privacy and dignity Be aware that the patient may have problems with swallowing. Ensure you maintain the patient's privacy and dignity. If an enema or suppository has been prescribed, ensure that privacy and dignity are maintained when administering the medication.

Position of patient Ensure the patient is in an upright position, to aid digestion.

Medication Ensure the medication is taken while you are at the bedside and not left for a later time.

Documentation Ensure a trained nurse signs for the drug in the correct place on the prescription sheet.

Report Report any problems, for example a patient refusing the medication.

Patient's comfort Ensure your patient is left in a comfortable position after administration of medication, and ask them if they require anything.

◼ OSCE SCENARIO: DRUG ADMINISTRATION

Read the scenario and then perform the skill of drug administration using the examiner as your second checker.

Mrs Jane Underhill is 80 years old and has been admitted with a chest infection. She is complaining of pain and a tickly cough. You are assisting on a drug round and have been asked by your mentor (a trained nurse) to show her the correct procedure for administrating Mrs Underhill's medication. Mrs Underhill has been prescribed 1 g of paracetamol and 10 ml of cough syrup, due at 8 a.m.

- Task to take 15 minutes – time yourself!
- Use the checklist below to practise the skill of drug administration

OSCE checklist: oral drug administration

SKILL	PERFORMED COMPETENTLY	PERFORMED BUT NOT COMPETENT	NOT PERFORMED/ INCOMPETENT
Communication: student introduces themselves and gains consent			
Examines drug chart for vital information, e.g. name, date, etc.			
Washes hands using Ayliffe procedure			

SKILL	PERFORMED COMPETENTLY	PERFORMED BUT NOT COMPETENT	NOT PERFORMED/ INCOMPETENT
Selects correct tablets/syrup			
Checks expiry date on tablets/syrup			
Calculates correct dose			
Uses non-touch technique to place tablets in pot; measures correct amount of syrup into a medicine pot			
Explains medication to patient			
Checks patient's identity against prescription sheet and arm band; checks other vital information, such as date, doctor's signature, route, amount, time, allergies and extra instructions			

SKILL	PERFORMED COMPETENTLY	PERFORMED BUT NOT COMPETENT	NOT PERFORMED/ INCOMPETENT
Ensures patient takes medication as prescribed			
Signs the drug chart with a qualified nurse			
Overall approach to task			
Pass/fail			

Scenarios for other branches of nursing

MENTAL HEALTH BRANCH

Mr Simon King has been admitted to hospital with anxiety and panic attacks. He has been prescribed diazepam 5 mg. You are the student nurse on duty and have been asked to administer Mr King's medication with the trained nurse.

CHILD AND YOUNG PERSON'S BRANCH

Miss Janet Fig is 15 years old and has been admitted with constipation. She has been prescribed 10 ml of lactulose. You are the student nurse on duty and have been asked to administer Jane's medication with a trained nurse.

LEARNING DISABILITY BRANCH

Mr Ernest Taylor is 35 years old and has asthma. He has been admitted with a mild asthma attack. Mr Taylor has been prescribed a nebuliser of 5 ml normal saline. You are the student nurse on duty and have been asked to administer the nebuliser medication with the trained nurse.

Useful websites

British National Formulary **www.bnf.org**
Department of Health **www.dh.gov.uk**
National Institute for Health and Clinical Excellence
   www.nice.org.uk
Nursing and Midwifery Council **www.nmc.org.uk**
Resuscitation Council **www.resus.org.uk**

Further reading

Baillie L (2005) *Developing Practical Nursing Skills*, 2nd edn. London, Arnold, 81–7, 214–15.

Bloomfield J (2010) *How to Pass Your OSCE: A Guide to Success in Nursing and Midwifery*. Harlow, Pearson Education.

Colbert B (2009) *Anatomy and Physiology for Nursing and Health Professionals*, Harlow, Pearson Education.

Davie A, Amore J (2010) Best practice in the measurement of body temperature. *Nursing Standard* **24**(42):42–9.

Department of Health (2006) *Essential Steps to Safe, Clean Care: Reducing Healthcare-Associated Infections. The Delivery Programme to Reduce Healthcare-Associated Infections (HCAI) Including MRSA*. London, Department of Health.

Department of Health (2003) *Winning Ways: Working Together to Reduce Healthcare-Associated Infection in England*. London, Department of Health.

Dougherty L, Lister S (2008) *The Royal Marsden Hospital Manual of Clinical Nursing Procedures*, 7th edn. London, Wiley-Blackwell.

Griffith R, Griffith H, Jordan S (2003) Administration of medicines: part 1. The law and nursing. *Nursing Standard* **18**(2):47–56.

Higgins D (2008) Specimen collection: part 3. Collecting a stool specimen. *Nursing Times* **104**(19):22–3.

McWilliam P, Botwinski I (2010) Developing a successful nursing objective structured clinical examination. *Journal of Nursing Education* **49**(1):36–41.

Resuscitation Council (UK) (2010) *Resuscitation Guidelines 2010*. London, Resuscitation Council (UK).

Small SP (2004) Preventing sciatic nerve injury from intramuscular injections: literature review. *Journal of Advanced Nursing* **47**(3):287–96.

Wallyniahmed M (2008) Blood pressure measurement. *Nursing Standard* **22**(19):45–8.

Waugh A, Grant A (2004) *Ross and Wilson's Anatomy and Physiology in Health and Illness*, 9th edn. Edinburgh, Churchill Livingstone Elsevier.

Final tips

Read and review	• Read and review anatomy and physiology related to each skill • Read and review each clinical skill procedure
Practise OSCE	• Individual practice • Group work – one student – one assesor – one patient
On the day	• Dress code – hair tied back and off shoulder – nursing flat shoes – fob watch – no jewellery – black pen • Stay cool, calm and collected

Good luck!

Shift roster

DAY	DATE	SHIFT
MONDAY		
TUESDAY		
WEDNESDAY		
THURSDAY		
FRIDAY		
SATURDAY		
SUNDAY		